Matters of Opinion

SMOKING

BY
PEGGY J. PARKS

NORWOODHOUSE PRESS
CHICAGO, ILLINOIS

Norwood House Press
P.O. Box 316598
Chicago, Illinois 60631

For information regarding Norwood House Press, please visit our website at:
www.norwoodhousepress.com or call 866-565-2900.

Paperback ISBN: 978-1-60357-582-9

The Library of Congress has cataloged the original hardcover edition with the following
call number: 2013051369

252N—072014
Manufactured in the United States of America in Stevens Point, Wisconsin.

Contents

Note: Words that are **bolded** in the text are defined in the glossary.

Timeline

1929 American doctor John Harvey Kellogg states that tobacco addiction is like opium or alcohol addiction.

1957 Surgeon General Leroy E. Burney states that smoking is one of the causes of lung cancer.

1959 The American Cancer Society links smoking to lung cancer.

1964 Surgeon General Luther L. Terry offers proof that smoking causes lung cancer, heart disease, and other serious health conditions.

1965 Congress passes the Federal Cigarette Labeling and Advertising Act. Tobacco companies must place health warnings on all cigarette packages sold in the United States.

1968 Seventy-eight percent of those interviewed in a Gallup poll think smoking causes cancer. Only 44 percent thought this in 1958.

1970 The Public Health Cigarette Smoking Act goes into effect and bans all ads for cigarettes on radio and TV.

1991 A study finds that kids six years old and younger recognize Joe Camel (of Camel cigarettes) as much as they do Mickey Mouse.

1993 The U.S. Environmental Protection Agency states that secondhand smoke causes lung cancer in adult nonsmokers and harms kids' lungs and breathing.

1994 In sworn testimony, the chief executives of the top seven tobacco companies say no evidence links smoking to cancer or other serious diseases. Less than one month later, confidential documents are discovered, showing that tobacco companies knew about smoking dangers as far back as the 1950s.

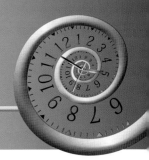

1997 The leading cigarette manufacturers and state's attorneys general announce changes in how tobacco products are promoted and sold in the United States. Cigarette makers must also pay tens of billions of dollars in damages over a period of time.

1998 Tobacco executives testify before Congress that nicotine is addictive and smoking may cause cancer.

2002 Delaware becomes the first U.S. state to enact comprehensive smoke-free legislation.

2009 Congress passes the Family Smoking Prevention and Tobacco Control Act. The law gives the U.S. Food and Drug Administration authority to regulate tobacco products the same way food and drugs are regulated.

2011 Of people who took part in a Gallup poll, 59 percent say they are in favor of smoking being banned in all public places, up from 39 percent in 2001.

2012 A study from the University of California–San Francisco shows that secondhand smoke kills 42,000 nonsmokers each year in the United States, including almost 900 babies.

2013 A study by the Harvard School of Public Health finds that graphic pictures and warnings on cigarette packages are much more effective at reducing smoking than words alone.

2014 CVS Caremark, the country's largest drugstore chain in overall sales, announces that it plans to stop selling cigarettes and other tobacco products by October.

1 Why Is Smoking an Issue?

Smoking used to be much more popular than it is today. In ads rugged cowboys sold Marlboro cigarettes. Pretty models told women to smoke Virginia Slims. Ads for Camel cigarettes had Joe Camel. This cartoon camel was on billboards for almost ten years. He was also in newspaper and magazine ads.

Even young kids knew Joe Camel. A 1991 study found that preschool kids recognized him right away. By the time kids were six years old, they knew Joe Camel as well as they knew Mickey Mouse. Health officials did not like this. They accused the company that made Camel cigarettes of trying to get kids to smoke. By 1997 Joe Camel was gone from all ads.

For nearly a decade the cartoon Joe Camel appeared on billboards and in newspaper and magazine ads. Public health officials shut down Joe Camel ads in 1997.

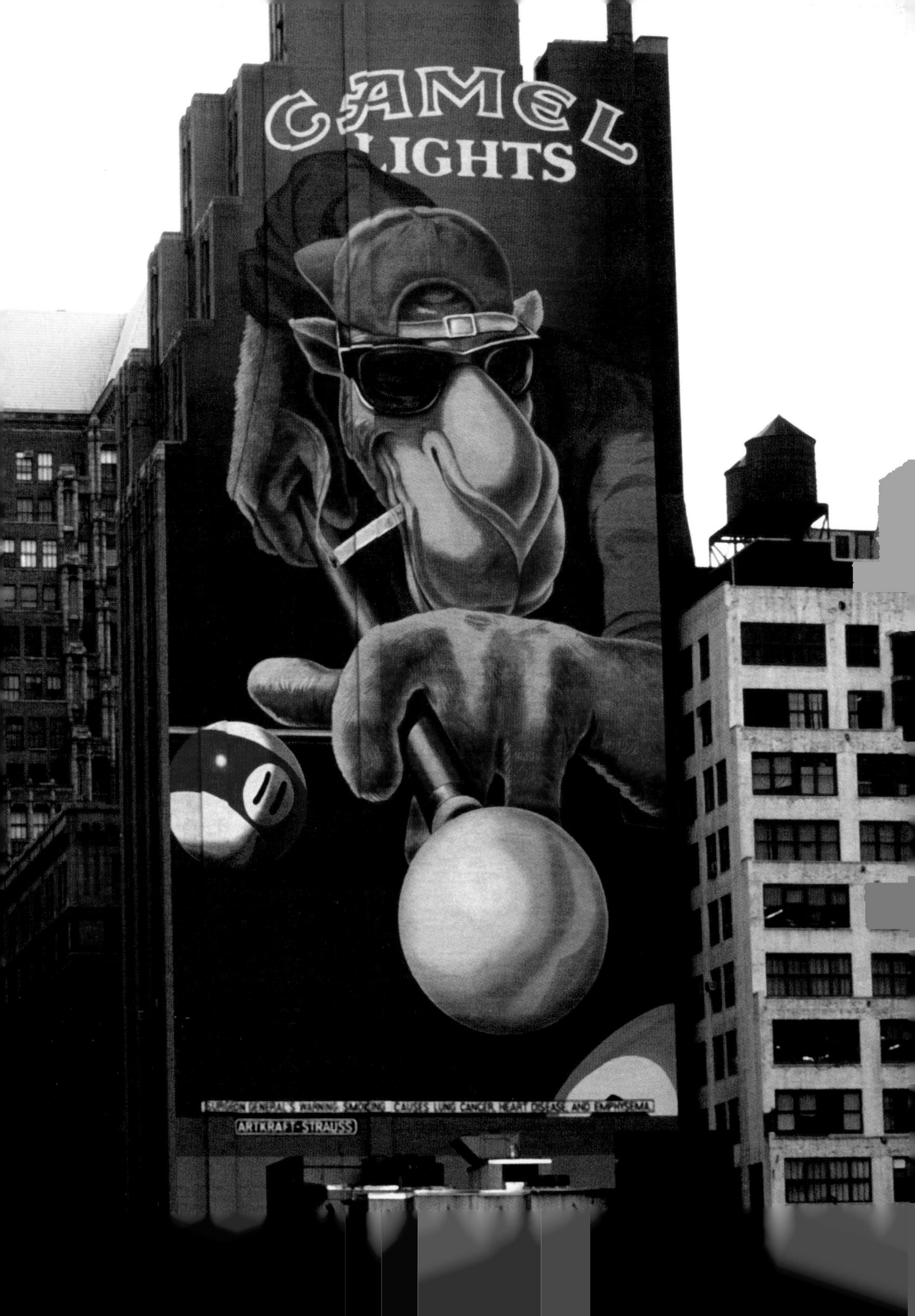
CAMEL
LIGHTS
SURGEON GENERAL'S WARNING: SMOKING CAUSES LUNG CANCER, HEART DISEASE, AND EMPHYSEMA
ARTKRAFT-STRAUSS

Every day, nearly 4,000 teens in the United States smoke their first cigarette, while 1,000 start smoking on a daily basis.

Health Damage

Smoking is no longer as popular as it was in Joe Camel's time. In recent surveys only about 20 percent of Americans say they smoke. That is much lower than the 1950s. Then, more than half of people smoked. Today people know much more about the dangers of smoking than their parents and grandparents did. Studies have shown that smoking harms health in many ways. When people hear about these findings, many choose to kick the habit.

The Centers for Disease Control and Prevention (CDC) did most of the studies on smoking. The CDC is the United States' leading health protection agency. Scientists who work there study smoking and health. "Smoking harms nearly every organ of the body," says

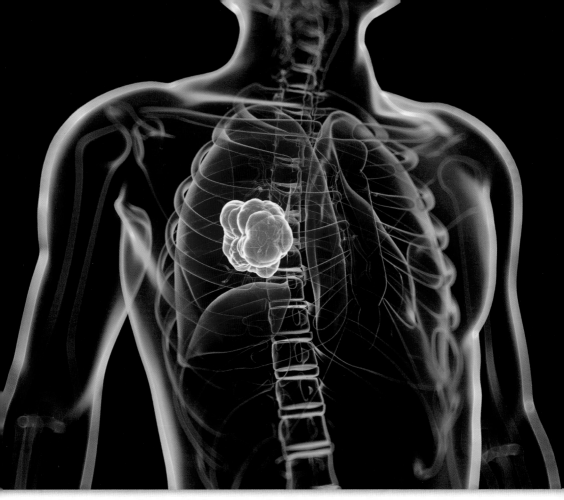

Computerized artwork showing a lung cancer tumor.

the CDC. "Smoking causes many diseases and reduces the health of smokers in general."[1] Smoking causes heart disease, **emphysema**, and lung cancer. Many other types of cancer have also been linked to smoking. These include leukemia (cancer of the blood), kidney cancer, bladder cancer, and stomach cancer, among others.

With all the health risks, people who do not smoke may wonder why smokers cannot just quit. But giving up smoking is not easy. Tobacco products have nicotine, which is very **addictive**. Smokers crave nicotine. Nicotine is so addictive that scientists say it is like hard drugs such as cocaine and morphine.

Shrinking Freedoms?

Few people deny that smoking harms the body. Even smokers often admit that. But smokers think it should be their own choice to smoke. This is at the heart of the smoking **controversy**. In the United States smoking is legal for people over the age of eighteen. If they can legally buy tobacco products, smokers think they should have the right to use them.

Beth Johnson has smoked for sixteen years. She is always polite to people who do not smoke. She never smokes when it might bother someone. Many times she has put out a cigarette for that very reason. But she feels that people are not always polite to her. "When you smoke, people treat you like you're evil or something!"

Robert Proctor is a science historian. He wrote a book called *Golden Holocaust: Origins of the Cigarette Catastrophe and the Case for Abolition*. In it he says that 6 trillion cigarettes are smoked every year. It is hard to imagine such a huge number. So Proctor explains it in his book. "[That's] enough to make a continuous chain from Earth to the sun and back, with enough left over for a couple of round trips to Mars.... Imagined as one long rod, that would be a cigarette more than 300 million miles long."

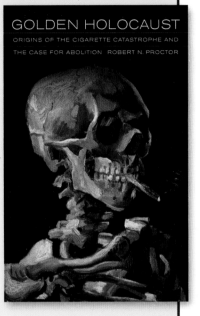

GOLDEN HOLOCAUST
ORIGINS OF THE CIGARETTE CATASTROPHE AND
THE CASE FOR ABOLITION   ROBERT N. PROCTOR

Robert Proctor, *Golden Holocaust: Origins of the Cigarette Catastrophe and the Case for Abolition.* Berkeley and Los Angeles: University of California Press, 2012, p. 3.

says Johnson. "And that's just wrong. If I'm not hurting you, or my smoke isn't anywhere near your face, why don't you just let me be? It's rude and **discriminatory** and I'm sick of it."[2]

Many smokers feel the same way. Although they can legally buy cigarettes, the number of places where they can smoke is shrinking. This is because most states have passed antismoking laws. As of August 2013, 36 states have some kind of law that restricts smoking in certain buildings. In addition to state laws, a growing number of cities and towns are passing local laws. New York City, for example, is known for its get-tough approach to smoking. People in New York are not allowed to smoke in restaurants, bars, workplaces, or many other buildings. As of July 2013 the American Nonsmokers' Rights Foundation says that 3,888 places in the United States have passed laws that restrict smoking.

Protecting Nonsmokers

Those who support strict antismoking laws are trying to protect the health of people who do not smoke. Their

Did You Know

Every cigarette you smoke reduces your life span by 11 minutes.

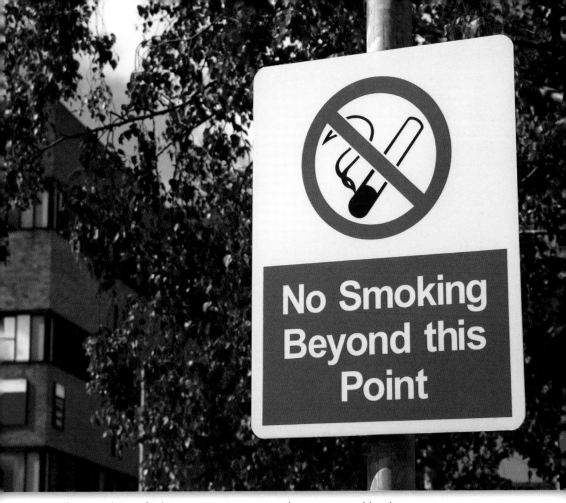

The number of places permitting smoking is steadily decreasing.

main concern is secondhand smoke. People who breathe in this smoke take **toxic** chemicals into their lungs just as smokers do. Dozens of studies have proved this smoke causes disease. One of these studies was released in September 2012. Researchers from the University of California–San Francisco found out something shocking.

They said secondhand smoke kills 42,000 nonsmokers in the United States each year. Almost 900 of those deaths are babies.

Going Too Far?

Such news causes many people to want even tougher laws. They think people should never get a whiff of smoke even if they are outside. This has led to outdoor smoking bans. In February 2011, for instance, smoking was outlawed at all New York City parks, beaches, and pedestrian plazas. California, Minnesota, and New Jersey have passed similar laws.

Many smokers resent these laws. Even some people who do not smoke have spoken out against such laws. One person who objects to them is Arthur L. Caplan. He is with the NYU Langone Medical Center. Caplan says there is no proof that outdoor smoking harms nonsmokers' health. So he thinks that laws banning smoking in outdoor areas are not needed.

A Cowboy's Change of Heart

In the 1970s Wayne McLaren was one of the most famous cowboys in the world. He was a Marlboro man. He was known for his rugged good looks and white Stetson hat. For 25 years he smoked up to two packs of cigarettes per day. But by the time he was 50, he regretted ever starting to smoke in the first place. McLaren developed lung cancer and died in July 1992. In an interview before his death, he said: "I'm dying proof that smoking will kill you."

Quoted in John Marchese, "A Rough Ride," New York Times, September 13, 1992.

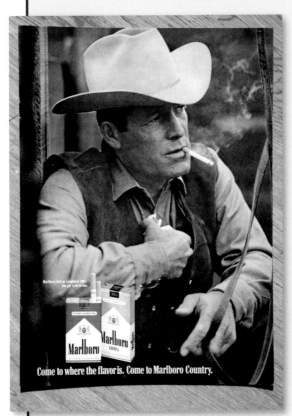

Wayne McLaren

While they may look like white cotton, cigarette filters are made of very thin fibers of a plastic called cellulose acetate. A cigarette filter can take between 18 months and 10 years to decompose.

A Look Inside This Book

In this book, three of the issues will be covered in more detail: Should people have the right to smoke? Should smoking be banned? Are tobacco companies responsible for smoking-related health problems? Each chapter ends with a section called **Examine the Opinions**, which highlights one argumentative technique used in the chapter. At the end of the book, readers can test their skills at writing their own essay based on the book's topic. Notes, glossary, a bibliography, and an index in the back provide additional resources.

2 Should People Have the Right to Smoke?

 Yes: People Should Have the Right to Smoke

When people talk about rights, they can mean different things. Americans often refer to rights granted by the Constitution. Free speech is one of those rights. With the issue of smoking, people speak about the right to make their own choices. Smokers claim that their right to smoke is being taken away by smoking laws. In cities and towns in the United States, people are allowed to light up in fewer places. Tony Newman works for the Drug Policy Alliance. "In some cities," he says, "it is nearly impossible to smoke anywhere besides your own home."[3] People legally have the right to smoke. But smoking bans have taken away their opportunities to do so. Many smokers say that is a form of discrimination.

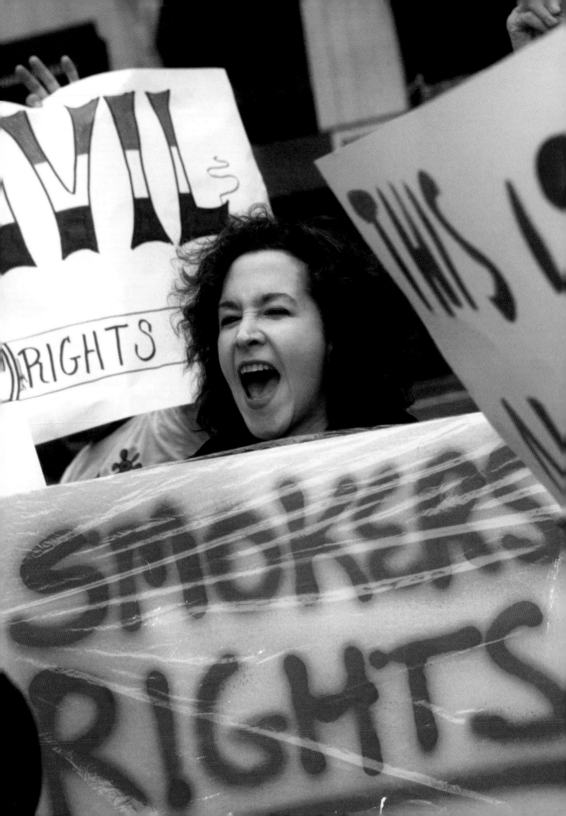

Smokers' Rights Taken Away

One city that is unfriendly to smokers is Charleston, South Carolina. Since 2007 smoking has been banned in restaurants and bars. It is also banned in workplaces. In 2012 the city council approved a new law. It restricted smoking even more. People can no longer smoke in a large area of downtown. This includes outside. For several blocks around a medical university and hospital, smoking is banned on public sidewalks and streets. Even people sitting inside parked cars are not allowed to smoke.

Writer Brian Hicks thinks such laws are much too strict. "We might as well go out now and change the city-limits signs. 'Welcome to Charleston—unless you're a smoker.'" Hicks and others who share his views think that smokers are being treated unfairly. He says that in Charleston smokers' rights have been taken away, and nonsmokers' rights are treated as more important. "And that's just wrong," says Hicks. "When did the rights of one group start to outweigh another's?"[4]

Many smokers say that smoking bans are a form of discrimination.

"The Dirty People"

Citizens Freedom Alliance fights for smokers' rights. Michael McFadden is one of its directors. He thinks that people who smoke are being treated unfairly. "It's like smokers have become the dirty people, and we don't want to see them," he says. "If they want to (smoke), they have to do it behind the dumpster.... It's gone way overboard."

Quoted in Joe Lawlor, "Maine Smoking Bans a Drag, or a Breath of Fresh Air?," *Portland (ME) Press Herald,* June 10, 2013.

Schools Toughen Rules

Hundreds of colleges and universities also have strict no-smoking rules. According to Americans for Nonsmokers' Rights, more than 800 colleges and universities are now 100 percent smoke free. One of them is Auburn University in Alabama. The ban was phased in slowly. This was to let students and employees have a chance to get used to it. At first smoking was banned within 25 feet (7.6m) of any building. By the fall of 2013, smoking

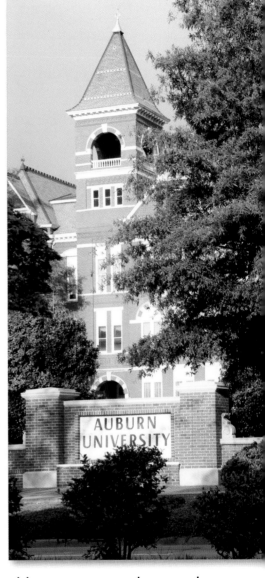

Auburn University banned smoking on campus in 2012. More than eight hundred college campuses across the nation are now smoke free.

was not allowed anywhere on campus. When the ban first started, many people were not happy. Smokers felt that their rights were being taken away.

In November 2012 George Washington University said it planned to ban smoking. Some people decided to protest the ban. A large group of students gathered in a campus plaza and chain-smoked for hours. Two of the students wrote a letter against the ban. "Smokers, though they may not like it, can understand the ban of smoking indoors," they wrote, "as the smoke remains in an enclosed environment, and those who do not like torched-tobacco cannot avoid it. Nonetheless, to now kick smokers out of outside...destroys the basic freedom of everyone."[5]

But Not So Fast...

 No: People Should Not Have the Right to Smoke

People who do not smoke think their point of view is just as important as that of smokers. They think that it comes down to an issue of health. When debating the smoking issue, people who do not smoke often quote Zechariah Chafee. He became well known for speaking of people's rights in a very simple way. He said that for every person with a personal right, someone else had a right to not be harmed by the possible consequences.

Chafee told of a man who was arrested after he swung his arms around wildly and hit another man in the nose. In court the man said that this was a free country. And he asked why he did not have the right to swing his arms around. The judge replied: "Your right to swing your arms ends just where the other man's nose begins."[6]

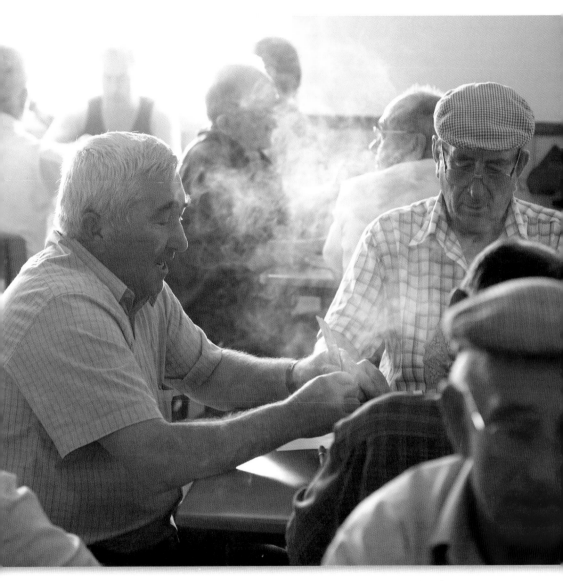

It has been proven that secondhand smoke increases the risk of cancer, heart disease, emphysema, and many other life-threatening diseases.

Breathing Rights

Chafee was not talking about smoking. But his words could apply to the smoking controversy. People who do not smoke think they are the ones being hit in the nose. Michaela Thurston is a student at the University of Alabama. She wrote a letter to the school newspaper. In the letter she called for stricter smoking rules on campus. She agreed that smokers have the right to

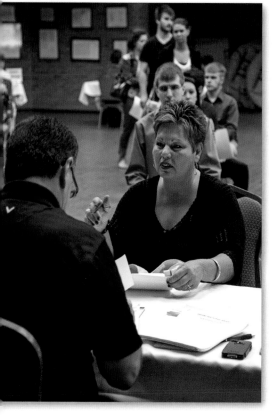

smoke. But she argued that those rights are not more important than the rights of people who do not smoke. She said: "Yes, an individual has the freedom to harm his or her own body, but that individual does not have the right to force similar harm upon another."[7]

Many companies today offer "Quit Smoking" programs as an employee benefit.

Colleges Should Be Smoke Free

According to the organization nosmoke.org, banning cigarettes on college campuses is justified. They argue that college-aged smokers have no right to smoke on campus because:

- *The majority of the U.S. population does not smoke.*
- *49.1% of the U.S. population is protected by a 100% smokefree workplace, restaurant, and bar law.*
- *Most local and state laws do not include college campuses, although some states do include state schools in their smokefree workplace laws....Therefore, there is a need to protect employees and students from exposure to secondhand smoke on college campuses and create an expectation that this living and working environment be smokefree.*

The organization also argues that by offering a smoke-free environment during the years when young people are most likely to take up the habit, colleges can prevent students from ever starting to smoke.

Thurston argued that secondhand smoke harms those who do not smoke. This means that smoking should not be allowed. It has been proven that secondhand smoke increases the risk of many life-threatening diseases

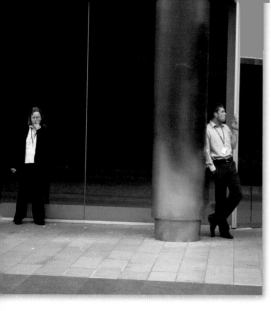

Nonsmokers believe their right to clean air is violated when people are allowed to smoke in public areas.

such as cancer. These also include heart disease and emphysema. According to the CDC, infants and kids who breathe this smoke are at risk for severe asthma attacks, breathing problems, and ear infections. The CDC writes: "There is no risk-free level of exposure to secondhand smoke."[8]

Closing Arguments

In the smoking debate, tempers often fly when the issue of rights is discussed. Smokers think that since smoking is legal, they should have the right to smoke. In their opinion, strict rules and laws limit their rights. Antismoking groups feel differently. They think restricting smokers' rights is the only way to protect the health of those who do not smoke.

Examine the Opinions

The Slippery Slope

A main idea found in this chapter is whether laws that limit smoking harm people's rights. Both smokers and nonsmokers argue that their rights are violated. Those who do not smoke think their right to clean air is harmed when people smoke in public areas. Smokers think their right to smoke is harmed when limits are placed on where they can smoke.

People who say that smoking is a right use several arguments to back up their belief. When looking at this issue, it is important to be able to recognize these techniques. Learning to identify some argumentative techniques can help you see whether an essay is based on facts or a person's opinion. Voicing an opinion is not wrong. But understanding what an argument is based on is important in order to better understand the material in this book.

When talking about smoking rules on campus, the author quotes a student who uses a **slippery slope** argument. This is when someone argues that something is wrong because it can lead to something worse, even though there is no proof that it would do so. When the student says, "To now kick smokers out of outside… destroys the basic freedom of everyone," she is arguing that one action is leading to a much worse action—the destruction of everyone's freedom. Clearly, the action of denying smoking on campus will not lead to the destruction of all students' freedom.

3 Should Smoking Be Banned?

No: A Smoking Ban Would Not Work

Many argue that the U.S. government should ban smoking. Others argue that such a ban would not be possible to police. These people often speak of Prohibition to prove their point. This was a law passed in 1919. It made alcohol illegal in the United States.

At the time, many people thought alcohol was a huge health problem. Those who favored Prohibition wanted to reduce Americans' alcohol use. But the ban made the problem worse. Once alcohol was banned, criminals sold it illegally. This was known as bootlegging. Alcohol sales did not slow down, they soared. So did crime. Congress realized its mistake, and in 1933 the law came to an end.

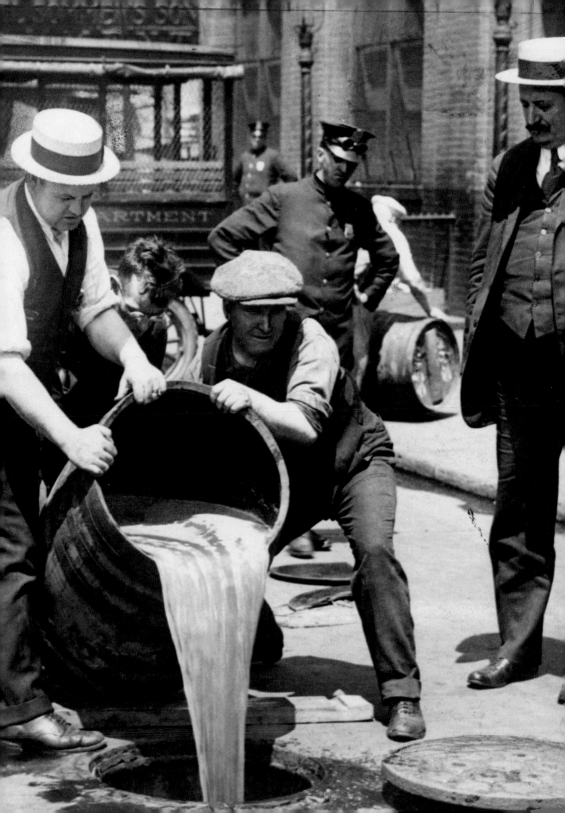

"Smoking in Alleys and Dark Corners"

Many people think the same thing would happen if smoking were banned. They say a ban would not keep people from smoking. Tony Newman agrees. He works for the Drug Policy Alliance. He thinks a huge number of people who now smoke would keep smoking anyway. He writes: "We would have smokers hiding their habit and smoking in alleys and dark corners, afraid of being caught using the illegal substance. We would have cops using precious time and resources to hassle and arrest cigarette smokers."[9]

Smokers could still buy tobacco products. They could buy them on the internet from other countries. There are billions of websites on the internet. It is not possible for U.S. officials to keep track of them all.

Beer is poured into a drain during Prohibition. Many see a correlation between prohibition of alcohol and the prohibition of smoking.

Smoking Banned?
What Comes Next?

Many people are against bans on smoking outside. They think that would take things too far. Dominic Dezzutti is a TV producer. He has looked into this issue. He thinks such bans take away people's civil rights. "We have already seen New York City attempt to ban large sodas," he says. "How long will it be before restaurants who serve fatty food are charged a 'health tax' to help subsidize health care costs? For that matter, with the amount of pollution that single drivers put in our collective atmosphere, why won't they be asked to pay more at the pump?" Dezzutti adds that these ideas may not be as far-fetched as they sound. "Smoking bans sounded ludicrous to us less than a generation ago, so be careful what you consider crazy."

Dominic Dezzutti, "Smoking Bans: When Will Simply Smoking Be Illegal?," CBS Denver, August 20, 2013.

Not the Government's Place

There is another issue with a complete smoking ban. It would harm people's civil rights. It is not the government's

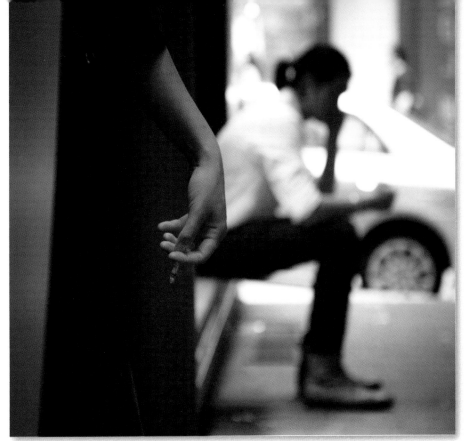

If smoking were banned, many people argue, it would not keep smokers from smoking.

place to try to protect people from themselves. Tom Head is a civil rights expert. He says it makes no sense to pass laws that restrict actions that harm people's health. Lots of actions that harm health are not banned. Head writes: "We may as well pass laws prohibiting people from eating too much, or sleeping too little, or skipping medication, or taking on high-stress jobs."[10]

But Not So Fast...

Yes: Smoking Should Be Banned

Those who support a smoking ban say that people's civil rights should be upheld. Their argument is that the U.S. government has passed many laws that make things illegal. Drugs such as marijuana, LSD, opium, and heroin are banned. People who support a smoking ban say the same principle could apply to smoking.

Tom Head says a smoking ban would not violate the Constitution. He points to past decisions by the U.S. Supreme Court. If a ban were put in place and the law were challenged, he thinks that the court would uphold the ban.

Growing Public Support

According to a July 2013 Gallup poll, public support for a federal smoking ban has been growing. More than 2,000 adults from all 50 states took part in the poll. One

Americans Say "Yes" to Car Smoking Ban

Many people do not want a complete ban on smoking. But they do want laws that protect kids from secondhand smoke. This was clear in a July 2013 poll by the C.S. Mott Children's Hospital. The poll surveyed 1,996 adults. Of these, 82 percent said they support a ban on smoking in cars when kids under 13 are in the car. Dr. Matthew M. Davis headed the survey. He says: "Smoke is a real health hazard for kids whose lungs are still developing, and especially for kids who have illnesses like asthma where the lungs are particularly fragile and flare up when exposed to secondhand smoke."

Quoted in Mary Masson, "82 Percent of Adults Support Banning Smoking When Kids Are in the Car," news release, UofMHealth.org, July 22, 2013.

question asked whether smoking in this country should be made totally illegal. Twenty-two percent said that it should.

That is less than one-fourth of the people who took the poll. This may not seem like a large number of people. But that 22 percent was a lot higher than in past surveys. In

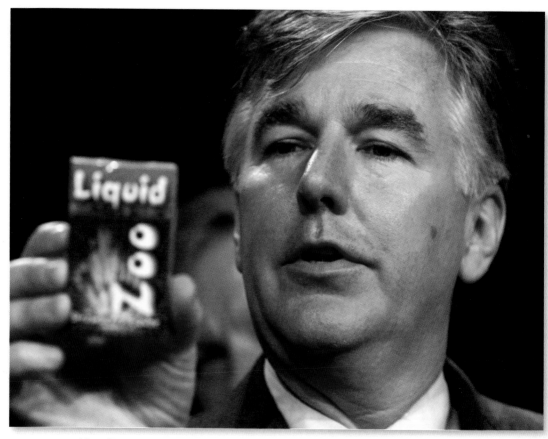

Health officials and politicians have come together to ban flavored cigarettes (pictured here), which they say lead teens to start smoking.

a 1994 Gallup poll, just 11 percent favored a smoking ban. When the new poll was released, a Gallup news release stated: "More Americans than ever want to ban smoking outright."[11]

Though a federal ban on smoking has not yet been enacted, many states have considered smoking bans.

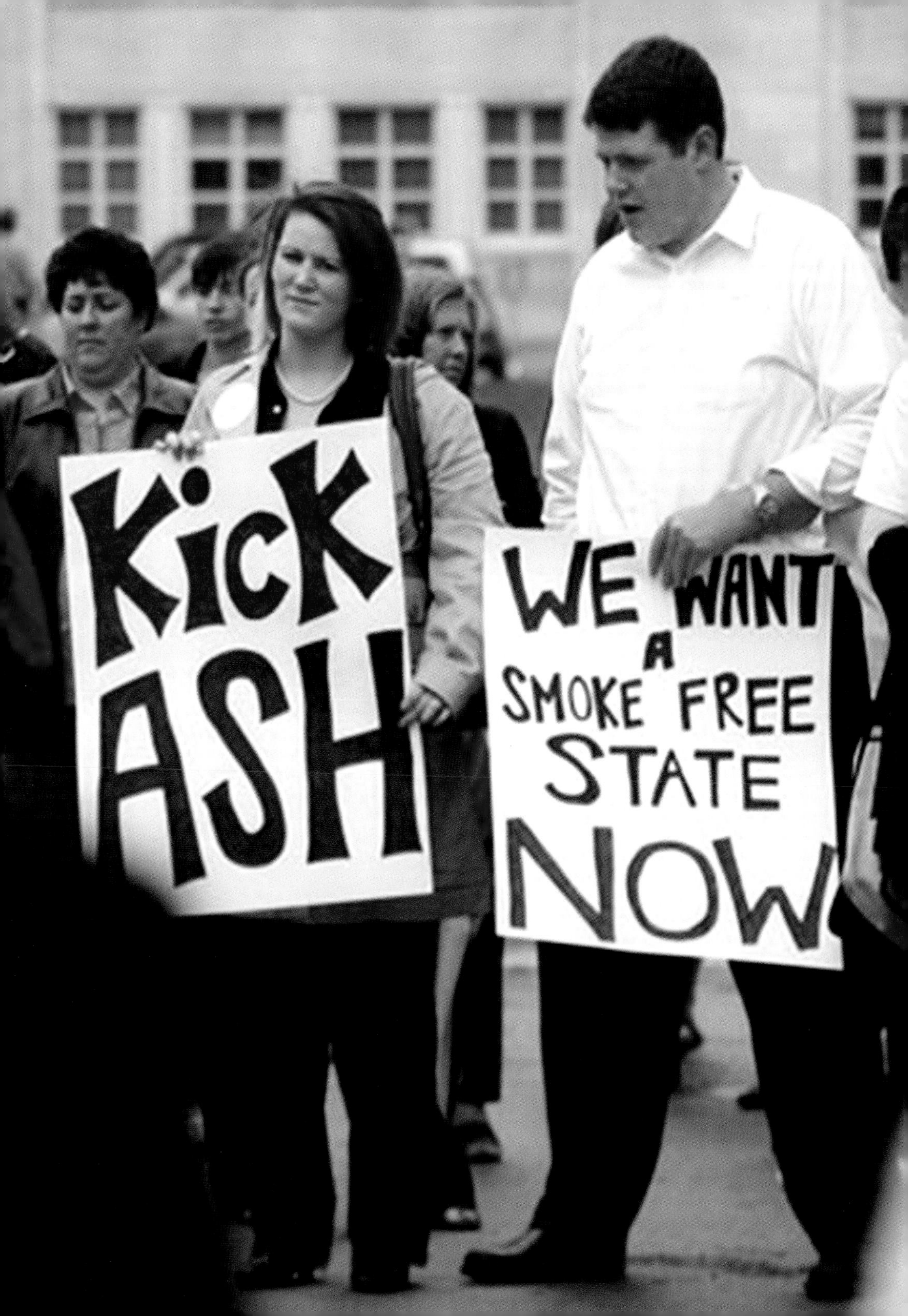
Kick ASH
WE WANT A SMOKE FREE STATE NOW

This is because most people think that smoking is a danger to health. This includes secondhand smoke. Whereas drinking alcohol does not usually harm people around the drinker, smoking can harm other people nearby. People who simply breathe the smoke can become sick. Some states are already thinking about a complete smoking ban. In 2013 Oregon introduced a bill that would make cigarettes illegal to buy without a doctor's prescription. But a doctor would probably not prescribe smoking. So the law would in effect ban cigarettes. The law is unlikely to pass. But it shows that some states are thinking about a complete ban.

Closing Arguments

Smoking is known to be dangerous. It causes many health problems. Even so, banning it would create a huge challenge. About 50 million Americans are smokers. For the government to take away their freedom to smoke would cause anger and resentment. To date, the U.S. government has not chosen to impose a ban.

Examine the Opinions

Scare Tactics

One argumentative technique is called a **scare tactic**. This is when the author makes frightening conclusions without really proving his or her point. In the first part of this article, the author quotes Tony Newman. He says, "We would have smokers hiding their habit and smoking in alleys and dark corners, afraid of being caught using the illegal substance. We would have cops using precious time and resources to hassle and arrest cigarette smokers." The author is using the example of the Prohibition era, when the United States banned alcohol. People had to sneak around to drink alcohol. Prohibition was repealed because it did not work. It did not stop anyone from drinking. This is just what happened during Prohibition to drinkers. The author's conclusion seems rational, even though the conclusions of a cigarette ban may be playing on people's fears.

When looking at author evidence for a viewpoint, it is a good idea to think about whether the conclusions seem logical or overly exaggerated. It is a fact that the United States tried to ban alcohol in the past and that it failed. But it is the author's opinion that a similar ban on smoking would create the same situation. It is important to understand the difference between a fact, which cannot be argued, and an opinion, which is one person's view of an issue.

4 Are Tobacco Companies Responsible for Smoking-Related Health Problems?

 No: Tobacco Companies Are Not Responsible for Smoking-Related Health Problems

On April 14, 1994, Congress held a hearing in Washington, D.C. Its goal was to look into health problems caused by smoking. Officials from the seven leading tobacco companies were at the hearing. One by one the officials denied that smoking caused lung cancer and other diseases. They said this had never been proven.

A few weeks later boxes of documents showed up at city offices. The sender was called himself "Mr. Butts." The documents traced back nearly forty years. They showed that the tobacco companies knew about

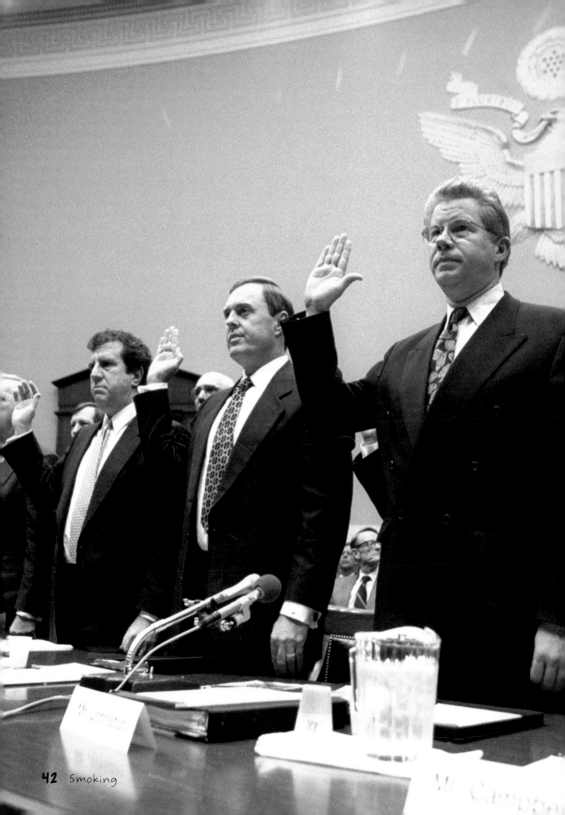

the risks of smoking. Company officials also knew how addictive nicotine was. It was clear that the tobacco officials had lied. The government forced them to pay billions of dollars in fines.

Time to Move On

Over two decades have passed since those events took place. Yet some think that people, not tobacco companies, are to blame for smoking's health costs. Lorne Gunter is a journalist. He does not smoke and never has. In fact, he says, "I detest smoking." He argues that if people choose to smoke, that is not the fault of tobacco companies. "Yes," says Gunter, "their ads are effective at glamorizing smoking. True, they make smoking appear cool or manly or pleasurable. But the decision to smoke is the smoker's. The tobacco companies do not come into homes, put guns to the heads of the unwilling and force them to light up."[12]

In 1994 officials from the seven leading tobacco companies testified at the Congressional hearing on health problems related to smoking and each said there was no connection between cancer and smoking.

The Blame Game

Jeff Jacoby is a newspaper columnist. He thinks it is wrong to blame tobacco companies for health problems caused by smoking. "The urge to blame others for our own self-destructive choices is as old as the power to choose," he says. Jacoby thinks this about adults as well as kids who smoke. He wrote of a woman who started smoking when she was thirteen years old and died of lung cancer in 2002. He said, "What turned her into a smoker was not a wicked corporation. It was a foolish choice she made as a teenager. People who willingly make foolish choices—a category that includes most human beings, especially those of the teenage persuasion—ought not to be enriched for their foolishness."

Jeff Jacoby, "Don't Fault Tobacco Firm for Death," *Boston Globe*, December 22, 2010.

Michael Kirsch feels much the same way. He is a doctor from Cleveland, Ohio. He saw the bad effects of smoking on people's health when he was a medical resident. "It kills people," he says. But he thinks that the blame for people's smoking is being unfairly pinned

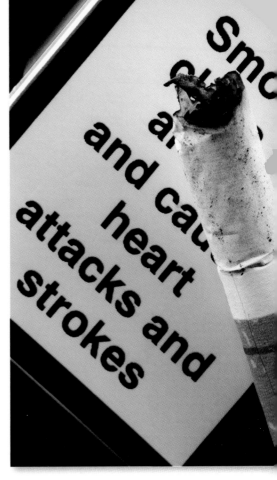

The fact that cigarette smoking was harmful to health was common knowledge even before cigarette warnings appeared on cigarette packages.

on tobacco companies. He writes: "This blame shift has always troubled me. I am well aware that the tobacco companies are guilty of many offenses.... My quarrel is blaming these companies for the decisions that individual smokers have made."[13]

Kirsch goes on to say that no one forces smokers to buy tobacco products. And they make the choice to smoke even though they know about the health risks. "Smokers for several decades knew...that cigarettes steal life and breath," he says. "This was common knowledge even before cigarette warnings appeared on cigarette packages."[14]

But Not So Fast...

James C. Salwitz sees things differently. Like Kirsch, he is a doctor. But Salwitz thinks smokers do not have total control over their decision to smoke. Yes, they freely choose to buy cigarettes and smoke. But Salwitz argues they do so because they are addicted to nicotine. "It makes no sense to blame the smoker for the behavior or the health consequences [that] follow," he says. "They are hooked junkie cigarette zombies."[15] There is no doubt in Salwitz's mind that tobacco companies are to blame for smoking-related health problems.

These companies make products that they know are addictive. According to Salwitz, that makes them the same as drug dealers. He calls nicotine "one of the most addictive chemicals known to man." He says it is more addictive than cocaine or heroin. Salwitz says

A Maddening Remark

Many people blame tobacco companies for health problems caused by smoking. They have different reasons for their beliefs. One is that the companies still will not admit how addictive cigarettes are. In May 2011 Louis Camilleri proved this to be true. He is the chief executive of Philip Morris International. At a meeting in New York, a cancer nurse spoke about one of her patients. The man had told her that he had beaten many drug addictions, including crack and cocaine. But he said cigarettes were the hardest to give up. Camilleri agreed that smoking is "harmful" and "addictive." But then

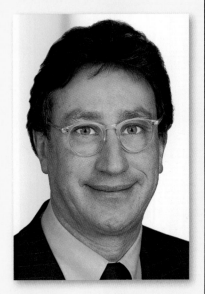

*Philip Morris's CEO
Louis C. Camilleri*

he said, "Nevertheless, whilst it is addictive, it is not that hard to quit." He was sharply criticized for what he said. So Philip Morris made a statement saying that tobacco products are addictive and harmful.

Quoted in Kathryn Kattalia, "Philip Morris CEO Tells Cancer Nurse: Quitting Isn't Hard for Smokers," *New York Daily News*, May 14, 2011.

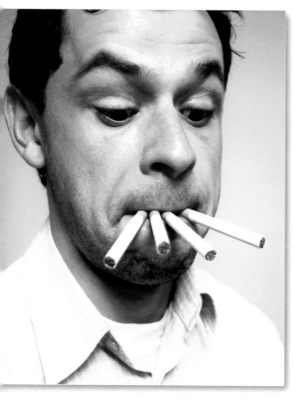

Addiction to nicotine keeps people smoking.

that changes occur in the addicted smoker's brain. When that happens the person is no longer able to make good choices. "This short-circuits free will," he says. Getting a "fix" by smoking, says Salwitz, becomes "almost as important to a smoker as food, warmth or even breathing."[16]

Addiction is a big concern for young smokers. Scientists know that kids' brains are not fully developed. This does not happen until they are in their twenties. When parts of a brain are still developing, it affects someone's ability to make good choices. So if kids decide to smoke, they cannot be held accountable in the

Too Young to Die

Laura Grossman was just 38 when she died of lung cancer. She started smoking as a teen. She smoked for 23 years. Her family blamed the R.J. Reynolds Tobacco Company. They said its ads were aimed at young people. They sued the company and won. In August 2013 a jury awarded the family $37.5 million. "The jury's message was loud and clear," says the Grossman's lawyer. "Big Tobacco should be protecting teens, not killing them. They should be curing cancer, not causing it. Instead, they continue to addict kids to nicotine, deliver these death sentences, and then try to blame smokers who they addicted."

Quoted in *Daily Mail* (London), "Tobacco Company Must Pay Lung Cancer Victim's Family $37.5 Million 'Because They Targeted Teens with Their Advertising,'" August 2, 2013.

same way adults can. The younger kids are when they start smoking, the more likely they are to get addicted.

Mixed Messages

Many people think tobacco companies try to get kids hooked. Robert Jackler is a professor of medicine at Stanford

University. He says, "Virtually all tobacco advertising is aimed at young people, and the reason is because almost nobody starts smoking beyond age 21 or 22."[17]

Critics say that tobacco companies pay to have ads in small stores near schools. These ads can lead kids to smoke. A 2012 report by the U.S. surgeon general says, "The more young people are exposed to cigarette advertising and promotional activities, the more likely they are to smoke."[18] Antismoking groups say that tobacco companies are not being responsible. They say this needs to stop.

Closing Arguments

Tobacco companies have been dishonest in the past. So they are often viewed as the bad guys. Years ago they made huge mistakes, and they paid a big price for it. Some people say that smokers make a choice and the responsibility is theirs. Others disagree. They think that tobacco companies deserve the blame because they still continue to make and sell addictive, harmful products.

Examine the Opinions

Testimonial

In this chapter the author quotes from two medical doctors who give opposing opinions about smoking. One doctor, Michael Kirsch, thinks that smokers are responsible for their health issues, not tobacco companies. He thinks that health choices—even poor ones—are a person's right and responsibility. On the opposing side, the author quotes another doctor, James C. Salwitz. He thinks that smoking is addictive. He argues that addicts cannot be wholly responsible for their actions.

When a writer quotes an authority in an article, it is called a **testimonial**. A testimonial is a good argumentative technique because it offers further proof of an opinion. In this case offering doctors' opinions is a good use of a testimonial. Doctors are qualified to offer health advice. But just because a testimonial is from a valid source does not mean that it is completely valid or without bias. Salwitz also says that smokers are "hooked junkie cigarette zombies" without free will. Such a statement is a biased opinion, even if it comes from a doctor. A reader needs to take into account that Salwitz has a view that addicts are not in control of their actions.

Wrap It Up!

Write Your Own Essay

In this book the author introduced many differing opinions about the issue of smoking. These opinions can be used as a launching point to write a short essay on smoking. Short opinion essays are a common writing form. They are also a good way to use the information presented in this book. The author presented several common argumentative techniques and evidence that can be used. In this book, slippery slope, scare tactics, and testimonials were presented as part of the essays to convince you. Any of these techniques could be used to enhance a piece of writing.

There are 6 steps to follow when writing an essay:

Step One: Choosing a Topic

When writing your essay, first decide on a topic. As a start you can use one of the three chapter questions from the table of contents in this book.

Step Two: Research Your Topic

Decide which side of the issue you will take. After choosing your topic, use the materials in this book to write the thesis, or theme, of your essay. You can use the articles and books cited in the notes and bibliography. You could also interview people in your life who are smokers or nonsmokers and quote them in your essay.

Step Three: The Theme

The first paragraph should state your theme. For example, in an essay titled "Smoking Should Be Banned in Public," state your opinion and what action you think should be taken to ban smoking and why. You could also use a short anecdote, or story, that gives an example of your point and will interest your reader.

Step Four: The Body of the Essay

In the next three paragraphs, develop this theme. To develop your essay, you should come up with three reasons why smoking should be banned. For example, three reasons could be:

- *Secondhand smoke has proven to be harmful.*
- *When someone smokes in a public place, others cannot avoid the smoke.*
- *Smokers do not have the right to harm other people's health.*

These three ideas should be developed into three separate paragraphs. Be sure to offer a piece of evidence in each paragraph. Your evidence could be a testimonial from a doctor or person who has been harmed by secondhand smoke. You could also use a scare tactic or a slippery slope argument to convince your reader of the urgency of the argument. Each paragraph should end with a transition sentence that sums up the main idea in the paragraph and moves the reader to the next.

Step Five: Writing Your Conclusion

The final, or fifth, paragraph should state your conclusion. This should restate your theme and summarize the ideas in your essay. It could also end with an engaging quote or piece of evidence that wraps up your essay.

Step Six: Review Your Work

Finally, be sure and reread your essay. Does it have quotes, facts, and/or anecdotes to support the conclusions? Are the ideas clearly presented? Have another reader take a look at your project in order to see whether she or he can understand your ideas. Make any changes that you think can help make your essay better.

Congratulations on using the ideas in this book to write a personal essay!

Notes

Chapter 1: Why Is Smoking an Issue?

1. Centers for Disease Control and Prevention, "Health Effects of Cigarette Smoking," Fact Sheet, August 1, 2013. www.cdc.gov/tobacco/data_statistics/fact_sheets/health_effects/effects_cig_smoking.

2. Beth Johnson, interview with the author, August 26, 2013.

Chapter 2: Should People Have the Right to Smoke?

3. Tony Newman, "Commentary: Why Not Prohibit Smoking?," CNN, July 30, 2009. www.cnn.com/2009/CRIME/07/30/newman.tobacco.ban.

4. Brian Hicks, "Charleston Is a Smoke-Free Facility," Charleston (SC) Post and Courier, January 10, 2013. www.postandcourier.com/article/20130110/PC16/130119937/1268/hicks-column-charleston-is-a-smoke-free-facility&source=RSS.

5. Ellis Klein and Christian Geoghegan, "Smokers of the World, Unite!," Scribd, November 13, 2012. www.scribd.com/doc/112889405/Smokers-of-the-World-Unite.

6. Zechariah Chafee, "Freedom of Speech in Wartime," Freedom of Speech, 1920, pp. 34–35.

7. Michaela Thurston, "A Right to Be Free from Smokers," letter to the editor, Crimson White, January 17, 2012. http://cw.ua.edu/2012/01/17/a-right-to-be-free-from-smokers.

8. Centers for Disease Control and Prevention, "Health Effects of Secondhand Smoke," November 15, 2012. www.cdc.gov/tobacco/data_statistics/fact_sheets/secondhand_smoke/health_effects.

Chapter 3: Should Smoking Be Banned?

9. Newman, "Commentary."

10. Tom Head, "Should Cigarettes Be Illegal?," About.com: Civil Liberties, 2006. http://civilliberty.about.com/od/drugpolicy/i/cigarettes_ban_2.htm.

11. Gallup, "In U.S., Support for Complete Smoking Ban Increases to 22%," July 29, 2013. www.gallup.com/poll/163736/support-complete-smoking-ban-increases.aspx.

Chapter 4: Are Tobacco Companies Responsible for Smoking-Related Health Problems?

12. Lorne Gunter, "Smokers Must Accept Consequences of Their Choice to Smoke," *National Post*, December 3, 2012. http://fullcomment.nationalpost.com/2012/03/12/lorne-gunter-smokers-must-accept-consequences-of-their-choice-to-smoke.

13. Michael Kirsch, "Stop Blaming Big Tobacco for Smokers' Decisions," MedCityNews, November 23, 2010. http://medcitynews.com/2010/11/stop-blaming-big-tobacco-for-smokers-decisions.

14. Kirsch, "Stop Blaming Big Tobacco for Smokers' Decisions."

15. James C. Salwitz, "Are Smokers to Blame for the Damage They Do to Their Bodies?," *KevinMD* (blog), May 12, 2012. www.kevinmd.com/blog/2012/05/smokers-blame-damage-bodies.html.

16. Salwitz, "Are Smokers to Blame for the Damage They Do to Their Bodies?"

17. Quoted in Jane Meredith Adams, "Despite Federal Ban, Tobacco Ads Continue to Lure Teen Smokers," EdSource, May 9, 2013. www.edsource.org/today/2013/despite-federal-ban-tobacco-ads-continue-to-lure-teen-smokers/31682#.Uj8vIiemU1I.

18. U.S. Surgeon General, "Preventing Tobacco Use Among Youth and Young Adults Fact Sheet," 2012. www.surgeongeneral.gov/library/reports/preventing-youth-tobacco-use/factsheet.html.

Glossary

addictive: A drug or other substance that, when taken, makes a person feel like he or she has no control over whether they use the substance or not. The person feels that he or she has to have that drug.

controversy: A subject that causes discussion, disagreement, or argument.

discriminatory: Relating to unfair treatment of one particular person or group of people. The treatment is usually related to someone's sex, religion, nationality, ethnicity (culture), race, or other personal traits.

emphysema: A lung disease most often caused by toxic chemicals or cigarette smoke. Emphysema breaks down lung tissue making it difficult to breathe.

scare tactic: A strategy that uses fear as a way of convincing someone of something.

slippery slope: Used in debate to argue that once something occurs, it will lead to a series of things that will be hard to control and will lead to worse events.

testimonial: A quotation used in support of a particular truth, fact, or claim.

toxic: Poisonous.

Books

Elizabeth Russell Connelly, *Nicotine = Busted!* Berkeley Heights, NJ: Enslow, 2006. In this book the author explores the many health risks of smoking and discusses the controversies associated with it.

Paul Mason, *Know the Facts About Drinking and Smoking.* New York: Rosen, 2010. This book presents the basic facts about smoking so young people can make good decisions and not get involved with substances that are harmful and addictive.

Articles

Jon Bush, "The Joys of Not Smoking," *Skipping Stones*, September/October 2012. The author of this article is an artist from Massachusetts. He used to smoke, and he says that quitting smoking is the best gift he could ever have given himself.

Nichole Buswell, "Clearing the Air: The Dangers of Occasional Smoking," *Current Health 2*, a *Weekly Reader* publication, October 2009. This article explains why smoking is always dangerous—even if someone only has a cigarette every once in a while.

Wendy Koch, "Graphic Ads Worked, CDC Says," *USA Today*, August 7, 2012. In this article readers learn how an ad campaign showing shocking pictures of smokers has been so successful that government health officials plan to do another campaign like it.

Crystal Phend, "Smokers' Kids Don't Get a Break in Cars," MedPage Today, November 12, 2012. www.medpagetoday.com/PrimaryCare/

Smoking/35878. This article talks about a disturbing study finding that most parents who smoke feel free to light up even when their kids are in the car.

Websites

It's My Life: Smoking (http://pbskids.org/itsmylife/body/smoking). With interactive features and games, this site educates young people about the hazards of smoking, the many toxic substances inside cigarettes, how to handle peer pressure, and comments from kids who were asked, "How do you feel about smoking?"

KidsHealth: Smoking Stinks! (http://kidshealth.org/kid/watch/house/smoking.html). On this website young people learn about the many health risks of smoking, how to help a parent who smokes, how to deal with peer pressure, and what other kids have to say about tobacco products.

Smoking Stinks! (www.smokingstinks-aaco.org). This site was created for kids by the Anne Arundel County Health Department in Maryland. It is chock-full of activities such as the Blast-a-Butt and Effects of Smoking games, a Chamber of Horrors that shows real pictures of diseases caused by smoking, a smoking quiz, and free downloads.

Index

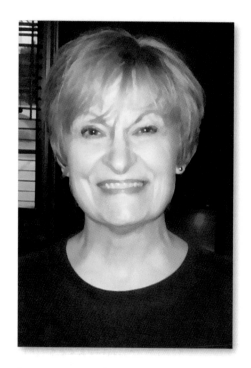

Peggy J. Parks holds a bachelor of science degree from Aquinas College in Grand Rapids, Michigan, where she graduated magna cum laude. An author who has written more than one hundred educational books for children and young adults, Parks lives in Muskegon, Michigan, a town that she says inspires her writing because of its location on the shores of Lake Michigan.